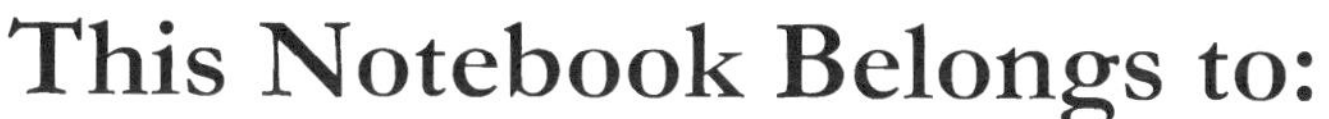

This Notebook Belongs to:

____

From Grief To Grind

Empowering grievers to heal their known and unknown grief and live a purposeful life.

www.fromgrieftogrind.co

Made in the USA
Columbia, SC
26 January 2025

aa0f9ce3-d454-4850-a8e1-afb69592811aR01